A DOCTOR'S GUIDE FROM
PANDEMIC
TO
NEW NORMAL

COVID PREVENTION, VACCINES, AND STRESS RELIEF

DOMINIC GAZIANO, MD

Distributed by Bublish Inc.

ISBN: 978-1647043-84-1 (Hardback)
ISBN: 978-1647043-86-5 (Paperback)
ISBN: 978-1647043-85-8 (eBook)

To all the caregivers, certified nursing assistants, licensed practical nurses, registered nurses, physicians assistants, nurse practitioners, physicians and other medical personnel who put aside their fears to tend to COVID patients in their time of need.

TABLE OF CONTENTS

INTRODUCTION

I AM DOMINIC GAZIANO, FONDLY called Dr. G, a practicing adult primary care doctor in Chicago. I've been constantly treating COVID patients since March 2020. I was on the front lines of the Chicago surge in March, April, and May of 2020. To remember is to tremble, and when I remember this horrifically dark and deadly period–the scariest and saddest time in my twenty years of practicing medicine–I tremble. With these images seared in my mind, I am motivated every single day to do my utmost to defeat this virus, and that motivation was the primary driving force for writing this book.

"The coronavirus was trying to suck the life out of me," one of my nurse colleagues told me. The day she came back to work after recovering from COVID, she related her horrific story to me. She motioned with her clasped hand, pulling it away from her chest, fully extending her arm outward, illustrating that the virus had been pulling the life out of her body during that time. A few weeks earlier, she had called me and said she was struggling to breathe and had a temperature of 104. I told her to go to the hospital immediately. Thinking that she might not make it, as she went into the hospital, she told her husband to take care of her children. She really believed it was the last time she would see her family. She spent five tumultuous days in the hospital, on oxygen, and went home to recover for a week.

She had difficulty breathing on and off and experienced weakness for about a month before she fully recovered.

I have witnessed the struggles that my hundreds of patients, young and old, and scores of health-care-worker colleagues have endured as a result of the virus. I saw how my nurse colleague went from being asymptomatic, or having no symptoms, to experiencing full-blown COVID in the hospital and in intensive care. Many have trouble comprehending this new reality, but I've seen these rapid progressions many times during the surge, and they are still occurring today.

A confidence that we could beat this immense and intense virus welled up inside of me. In September 2020, I heard that a COVID vaccine was on the horizon. A huge feeling of relief and urgency came over me. I knew I had to promote the vaccine and educate my patients on why they had to get it. I knew that this would be the thing that would save us. As a primary care doctor, I knew I couldn't live with myself in the years to come if I did not do this. Never in my medical career would I have an opportunity to do more good than I did now. I had to first calm the fears of my patients and then reinforce what they needed to do to keep themselves and their loved ones safe. I would explain to them that there were many ways to defeat this virus, and that they needed to do their part.

Through these hundreds of one-on-one conversations, I realized that people were mentally exhausted by COVID and, additionally, had heard so much confusing news and misinformation. They were still trying to sort out COVID and said they could not handle a heavy conversation about the vaccine. I had to get them out of their COVID disillusionment or downright paralysis and give them some hope that if we did the right things and got the COVID vaccine, we could get back to a new normal.

Given the gravity of COVID, it is important for all of us to reach out to informed medical professionals in order to better understand its difficult and scary concepts and then get on a cooperative path with the others in our community to put this pandemic to an end.

It is in this spirit that I write this book to logically work through your questions and to help you better understand the virus and the scientific solutions that medical professionals and scientists are building to help us all. We do have a solution to get back to a new normal in a matter of months. We must understand this as quickly as we can. This book is an attempt to explain some common concepts regarding the virus. Understanding these concepts well and practicing them will get you back to a new normal. In this book, I will put forth recommendations to achieve this new and better normalcy.

Over the course of this book, by using my intimate experience in fighting this virus, I want to increase your understanding of the truth about COVID, instill in you the belief that we do have a distinct pathway to defeat it, help address your fears regarding COVID, relate strategies to instill a sense of consistency in your daily routines from here on out, give you hope, and end this pandemic as quickly as possible. Finally, I will give a picture of a better post-COVID world.

I have had hundreds of conversations with patients in regard to their stress about COVID. For COVID fear and stress, I would counsel my patients in the same fashion as for other types of stress. I would get to the root cause of their stress. We would look at these causes logically and find a collective solution for how to cope with the stress. For COVID stress, I would add the additional step of trying to instill some hope that if we all do the correct things, then we can end this pandemic and get back to a new normal.

Starting at the beginning and going straight through the chapters to the end will provide the best understanding of the concepts in this book. However, feel free to jump around in order to find answers to some of the burning questions you may have about COVID.

There's a saying that "knowledge is power." In this case, knowledge and the proper understanding of COVID becomes the power to save lives. Over the last few decades, many have grown to distrust medical establishments. But we need to learn to trust them and their sound advice in regard to COVID. In the end, we must be able to discern sound advice for ourselves. We also need to know where to look for credible sources of information and how to implement some basic principles of interpreting the information. You will learn to do both of these things in this book. Once you understand these important COVID concepts, please practice them and pass them on in a "kumbaya" way so that we can end this pandemic.

1 UNDERSTANDING COV-2, THE CORONAVIRUS

"Nothing in life is to be feared; it is only to be understood. Now is the time to understand more, so that we may fear less."

–Marie Curie

THE CORONAVIRUS IS NOT GOING to stop–globally or in the US–until 60 to 70 percent of us have had it. The sad fact is that some of us react very poorly to this virus, while others recover with no lasting effects. Therefore, everyone should get vaccinated.

We are at war with this virus, and if we want to win, we must first understand the enemy. Allow me to explain our adversary and what makes it so formidable. At the end of this section, you will understand the parts of the virus that affect us, as well as those that are vulnerable to our interventions through means as simple as handwashing and other lifestyle habits. I will also explain how the virus can be deactivated through current and future vaccines.

THE CORONAVIRUS STRUCTURE

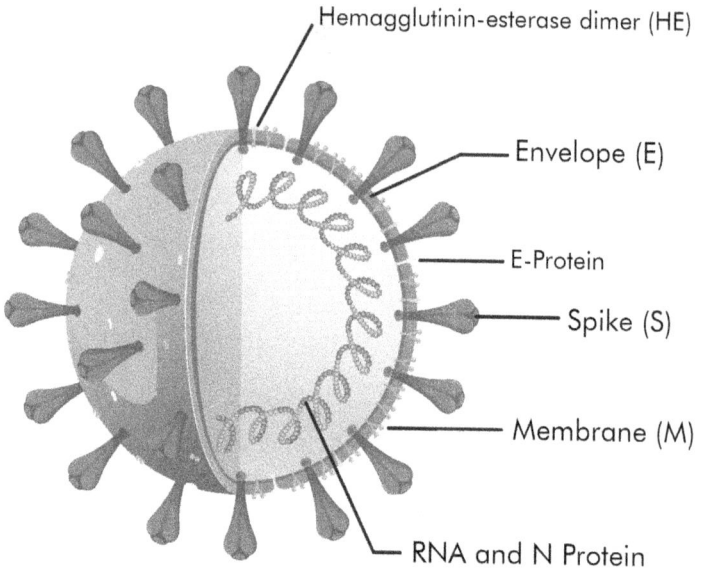

Hemagglutinin-esterase dimer (HE)

Envelope (E)

E-Protein

Spike (S)

Membrane (M)

RNA and N Protein

The diameter of a single coronavirus is equal to one one-thousandth of the width of a human hair. Many thousands of viruses are contained in a tiny water droplet expelled in a single cough or sneeze. These droplets can float in the air for extended periods of time and survive on a variety of surfaces. For example, it can live on metal for forty-eight hours, on plastic for seventy-two hours, and on cardboard for twenty-four hours. Hospitals typically use paper bags to hold reusable personal protective equipment (PPE) because of the virus's short lifespan on that material.

There are currently seven known coronavirus strains in the coronavirus family. Most are transmitted from human to human, but cats, bats, and other animals (mostly mammals) act as intermediary carriers in infecting humans.

THE CORONAVIRUS FAMILY

Human Coronavirus 229E	HCoV-229E	CAUSES COMMON COLD
Human Coronavirus 0C43	HCoV-0C43	
Human Coronavirus NL63	HCoV-NL63	
Human Coronavirus HKU1	HCoV-HKU1	
Severe Acute Respiratory Syndrome Coronavirus	SARS - CoV	CAUSES A DEADLY SYNDROME
Middle East Respiratory Syndrome Coronavirus	MERS - CoV	
Severe Acute Respiratory Syndrome Coronavirus	SARS - CoV-2	

In the above diagram, you can see that four of the seven coronavirus strains cause common-cold–like symptoms. Until 2002, these four strains were the only known coronaviruses. In November 2002, the first of three deadly coronaviruses was discovered in southern China. The first of these—the fifth in the list above, SARS-CoV or SARS-CoV-1—caused an atypical pneumonia, which was later identified as severe acute respiratory syndrome.

The second deadly coronavirus—sixth in the above list—is known as Middle East respiratory syndrome (MERS, or MERS-CoV). MERS is believed to have originated from bats and camels in the Arabian Peninsula, more specifically in Jedi, Saudi Arabia, and to have infected humans who had close contact with camels.

It should be noted that both SARS-CoV-1 and MERS are more deadly than SARS-CoV-2 (or COVID-19). There have been approximately 8,000 cases of SARS-CoV-1, around 9 percent of which were fatal. MERS has had about 2,500 cases, with an astonishing 35 percent fatality rate. Comparing this with the current approximated 2 percent mortality rate of COVID-19 in various countries, we can grasp the importance of containing an epidemic in its early phases, preferably in the area where it originated. With both the SARS-CoV-1 and the MERS viruses, aggressive measures were taken early in order to contain these deadly viruses before they became a pandemic. Spending effort and resources early on when numbers are small, tracking down every case to its origin, and making zero transmission the goal brings epidemics to a halt. The lesson is that we need to contain virus outbreaks in our cities early and bring transmission down to zero.

As for COVID-19, it is believed to have started in a wet market, that is, a place where live animals are brought in from other areas and sold. SARS-CoV-2 is believed to have originated in bats. Two mutations have since occurred; one of them made the virus in bats more infectious, and the second made the virus more deadly.

It is useful here to explain genetic transmission and wet markets. Wet markets are commonplace in Hong Kong and mainland China. A wet market typically sells live seafood, meats, and sometimes live animals that are kept in cages for long periods and interact with humans.

These live animals are typically brought in from rural provinces. They are under stress and live in captivity for long periods of time. Thus, genetic mutations occur in the animals, which can lead to viruses spreading more easily and can also make them more deadly. There has been pressure to outlaw wet markets because of the transmission of various viruses, bacteria, and other pathogens and organisms that can harm humans. This is called zoonotic disease transmission and is believed to be what caused the transmission of COVID-19 from animals to humans. The Chinese wet markets were shut down on January 1, 2020, because of the belief that SARS-CoV-2 may have been transmitted from animals to humans there.

THE ANATOMY OF THE CORONAVIRUS

Below is a list of various parts of the coronavirus:

RNA – the blueprint for proteins that the virus needs to reproduce itself.

Viral envelope – the outer layer used to anchor its structures and protect the virus.

Envelope proteins – proteins embedded in the viral envelope, which help put together the proteins after the virus has infected another cell.

Spike proteins – proteins projecting out and attaching to the host cell.

The coronavirus, like many other viruses that infect humans, uses human cells to replicate itself. This viral replication can destroy the human cells, which causes damage to the body and triggers an immune reaction to fight the virus. Both this virus invasion and the immune reaction are what make us sick.

At the core of viral replication is RNA, which is similar to DNA but does not need to enter the cell nucleus to reproduce. The RNA does not contain all of the genetic information of a cell. It contains genetic information for various viral component produced outside the nucleus.

The RNA sequence is used to code for components such as proteins and other structures in order to build more coronaviruses. The shell of the virus is made of a membrane that has been cannibalized from the previous host cell. The purpose of the membrane is to protect the interior RNA as well as to act as an anchor that holds the spike proteins and other elements of the virus in place.

The Coronavirus Entering our Cells

CORONAVIRUS

1. Coronavirus, or CoV with spike proteins, binds to a receptor on our body's cell

OUR BODY'S CELL

2. CoV enters our body's cells after fusing with our cell membrane

3. CoV internal viral RNA is released to the interior of our body's cells

4. The CoV uses our body's machinery to make new CoV proteins

5. Assembly of the CoV RNA and the newly formed proteins make a newly formed coronavirus

6. Vesicles fuse with the cell membrane and **release** CoV virions into the lumen

7. The newly formed coronavirus is released outside of our cells and goes off to infect some more of our body's cells

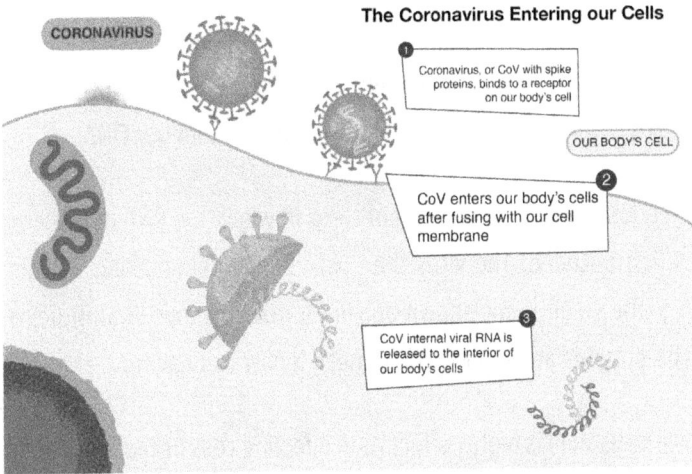

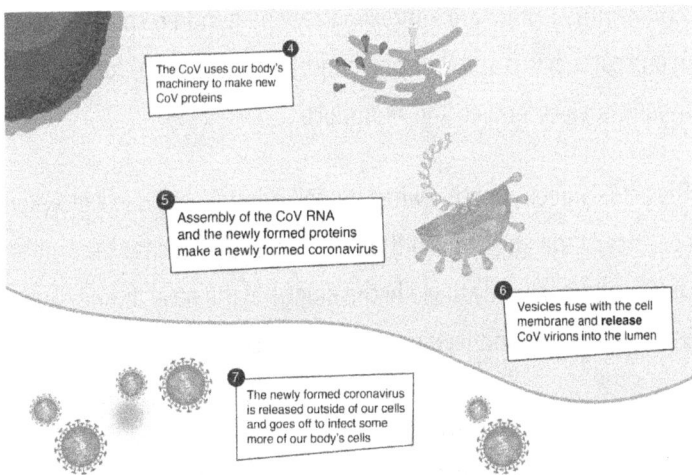

In the above diagram, you can see in step one how the coronavirus spike proteins attach to and then enter our cells. Note how the virus sidesteps the nucleus—shown as a big brown dot in the diagram. The

cell DNA is always housed in the nucleus. Sidestepping the nucleus means it's impossible for the virus to incorporate into our DNA. All vaccines for the coronavirus thus far also sidestep the nucleus and make it impossible to incorporate sequences into our DNA.

Step four represents a series of steps in which the RNA of the virus is first decoded. The virus then uses our protein-making machinery–the Golgi body, shown above–to make various viral proteins. The proteins are assembled to make a new coronavirus.

The virus shell is highly effective in infecting cells because of the "S" or "spike" protein. Some say it looks like a crown–hence the name "coronavirus." There are approximately one hundred spike proteins in one coronavirus and thus one hundred opportunities for the virus to infiltrate our bodies and reproduce.

The actual infection occurs when the spike protein binds to a receptor, specifically the angiotensin II receptor (ACE-2), which is present on many cells, especially those in the linings of the nose, throat, upper bronchial tubes, and lower respiratory tract.

Once the spike protein activates the receptor, changes occur in the proteins to allow the virus to get into the body's cells. Once inside the cell, the virus releases its RNA and uses the cell's protein-manufacturing body, the ribosome, to create proteins. The virus then reassembles these proteins into new virus strands, and the virus multiplies inside cells until they burst open, thereby continuing to spread itself.

There are two primary ways in which the coronavirus enters the body. First, when a person speaks, sings, or coughs, they send out water droplets, each potentially containing thousands or tens of thousands of coronavirus particles. The droplets can land on a person's skin and get into their nose, mouth, and eyes. The droplets can remain airborne for two to three hours, and so a person can be exposed long after an infected individual was present. If an individual is in a room where these tiny particles are present for more than fifteen minutes, they have a greater likelihood of infection.

The second way that the coronavirus enters the body is when one touches a surface that has been contaminated, with the virus residing outside the body on fomites. Fomites are objects made of various materials that the virus can survive on, including countertops and doorknobs. If a person touches a contaminated surface and then touches their face, the virus can get into their body. Some bacteria and viruses cannot live long outside a host, but coronaviruses have the ability to survive on fomites for varying lengths of time, hours to days, depending on the type of surface.

Thorough handwashing can inactivate the virus or remove it completely from your hands, thereby minimizing the chances of infection. You should always wash or sanitize your hands after touching surfaces in public places.

2 UNDERSTANDING HOW COVID AFFECTS THE BODY

"Sometimes you just have to die a little bit inside in order to be reborn and rise again as a stronger and wiser version of you."

— Aagam Shah

AS A NURSING HOME MEDICAL director, I was responsible for being available to the registered nurses, LPNs, and other nursing home staff as they developed fevers and other COVID symptoms. The COVID surge in the spring of 2020 wreaked havoc in the nursing homes that I served in Chicago. I sent three nurses and a cleaning staff member to the hospital, and fortunately they all had good outcomes. One of these three nurses relayed her severe symptoms in the same way as she would relay a patient's that we were taking care of together. I tell this story in the introduction of this book–how she was telling her family she might not make it. I came to understand on another level how COVID takes hold of and devastates our bodies and how it evokes the fear she described in her week-long battle in the hospital. In this chapter, I will share with you how

COVID affects our bodies, and in subsequent chapters, how COVID affects us emotionally.

In my experience diagnosing and treating hundreds of COVID patients, I have observed a wide spectrum of demographics and disease presentations. One of my patients was a twenty-eight-year-old woman who worked at a restaurant. She suffered from severe back pain, muscle aches, and weakness for three weeks before finally recovering. I had another very old patient in the nursing home, whom I sent to the hospital. She appeared to be turning the corner from severe COVID pneumonia, only to suffer a massive stroke and die. One of my colleagues in infectious diseases related a story of his medical coworker who ended up with COVID after a family gathering. She was hospitalized and died from severe COVID pneumonia within one week. The virus does not discriminate. Anyone is susceptible to chronic illness and even death from it.

I have witnessed my patients' and health-care colleagues' physical and emotional struggles with COVID. I have seen how quickly a patient can go from asymptomatic to full-blown COVID in the hospital–to the extent of requiring intensive care. Many people have trouble comprehending this new reality, but I have seen these rapid progressions of COVID illness scores of times, and they continue to this day.

In chapter 1, we reviewed the characteristics of the virus, how one can potentially contract it, and how it replicates on a cellular level in the body. In this section, we will discuss how coronavirus can cause illness throughout your body. We will review how it causes symptoms when it first enters the body, how it progresses, and how it can cause serious damage as the body fights the disease, along with the potential long-term medical complications.

One of the difficulties with COVID is that many people are asymptomatic for extended periods, during which they can still infect others. Those with asymptomatic COVID are infective for about a week on average but can be infective for up to ten days.

When the virus enters the body, it infects cells in the mouth, in the nose, and especially in the back of the throat. Initial symptoms include fever, shortness of breath, sore throat, and headaches. It should be noted that there are a variety of potential symptoms in addition to those listed above, such as abdominal pain, diarrhea, and confusion. The above are just some of the common symptoms. It is easier to diagnosis COVID if you have the more common symptoms of a dry cough, fever, or sore throat. Another pathway of entry for the coronavirus is the eyes. A small percentage of patients, perhaps 5 or 10 percent, have some ocular symptoms during the onset or over the course of the COVID disease.

However, you can have COVID with other less common symptoms, or no symptoms, so it's best to share your symptoms with your doctor and provide your exposure and testing history.

As the virus infects the throat, it produces a dry cough and sore throat. It may cause a low-grade or high fever, usually above 100.4. When the body's strong immune response kicks in, it can cause additional symptoms such as fatigue, confusion, and gastrointestinal problems like diarrhea, vomiting, and abdominal pain.

Studies conducted in the United States suggest that about 40 percent of COVID patients are asymptomatic, 40 percent have mild disease, 15 percent have severe disease requiring oxygen and likely hospitalization, and 5 percent are critically ill patients in intensive care who require ventilation.

More severe symptoms occur as the virus makes its way to the lower respiratory tract and bronchial tubes to the alveoli, which is where gas exchange occurs. Another area that can incur damage is the blood vessels. Clotting can occur anywhere in the body, not just in the lungs, and can lead to heart attacks, strokes, and kidney failure. Many patients experience loss of taste or smell. Most recover these senses after a couple of weeks, but some may lack taste and smell for up to two months. Finally, COVID can lead to long-term damage to our bodies, especially permanent lung injury and pulmonary fibrosis. There are other potential long-lasting symptoms, including neurological and other side effects, which are still being studied.

COVID severity is based on coronavirus viral shedding and viral load.

HOW CORONAVIRUS CAN SPREAD THROUGH THE AIR WITH A COUGH OR A SNEEZE

SINGLE SNEEZE CAN PRODUCE UP TO 10,000 DROPLETS.

SINGLE COUGH CAN PRODUCE UP TO 3,000 DROPLETS.

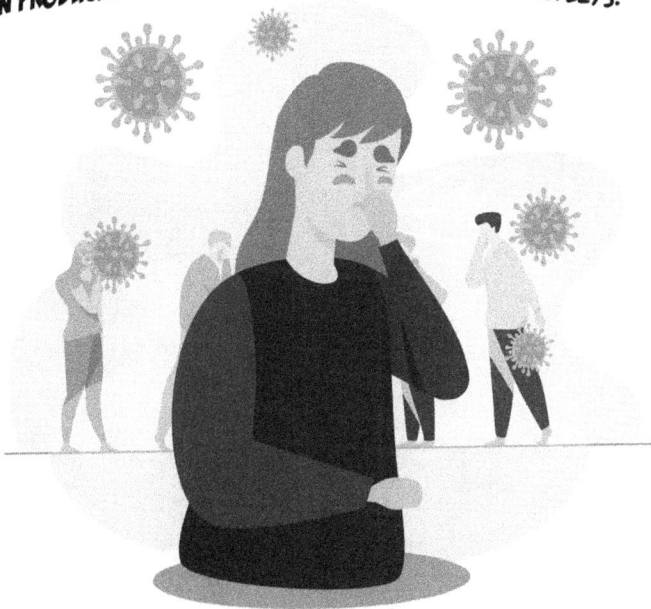

Viral shedding refers to how fast the virus can spread from one part of the body to another part of the body as well as how it spreads from our bodies into the environment. Viral shedding in closed spaces is more likely to result in human-to-human transmission.

Therefore, people should avoid being in nonventilated indoor spaces for longer than fifteen minutes.

HOW CORONAVIRUS CAN SPREAD THROUGH THE AIR WITH A COUGH OR A SNEEZE

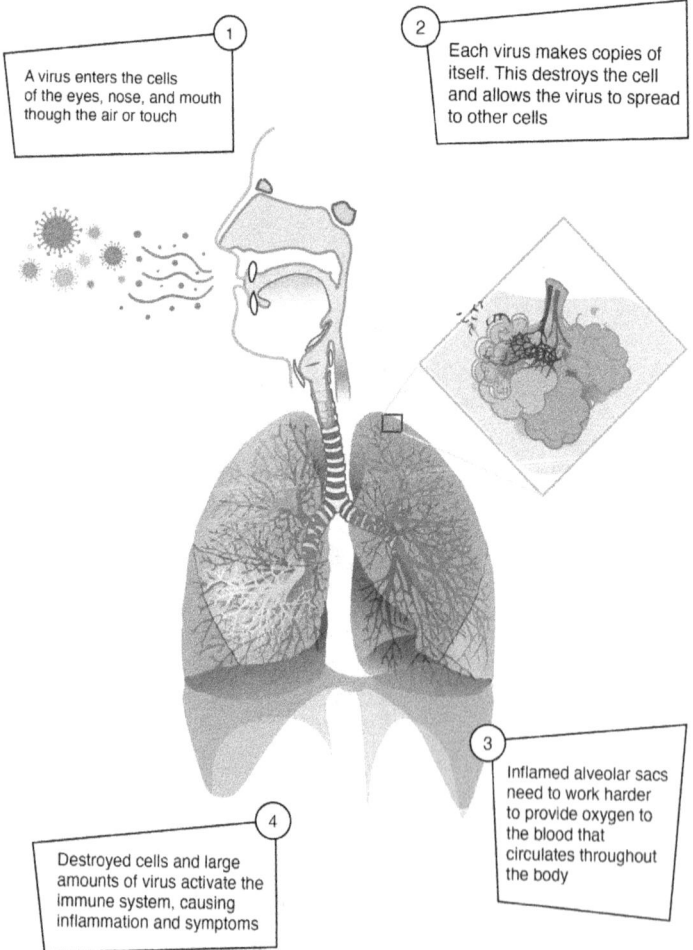

1
A virus enters the cells of the eyes, nose, and mouth though the air or touch

2
Each virus makes copies of itself. This destroys the cell and allows the virus to spread to other cells

3
Inflamed alveolar sacs need to work harder to provide oxygen to the blood that circulates throughout the body

4
Destroyed cells and large amounts of virus activate the immune system, causing inflammation and symptoms

If a person is near several infected others at once, that person will contract a greater viral load. The greater the viral load, the more severe the symptoms and potential organ damage, as both the viral invasion and the body's response will be more significant.

Viral load refers to the virus concentration in a patient's bloodstream, which is measured in virus particles per milliliter. Research shows that those who have been exposed to many infected individuals can contract a greater viral load and incur greater damage to their bodies. The more viral particles that come into the body at once, the greater the damage to our bodies. This higher concentration of virus, or viral load, will elicit a much stronger immune reaction, or "cytokine storm." Our normally helpful cytokine chemicals, combined now with COVID, produce a damaging effect on our organs, resulting in multiple areas of inflammation. Other viruses, such as influenza, are localized to one area of the lung or lobe and do not spread so quickly through the lungs and other organs.

Inflammation, in regard to a viral infection, is usually triggered by damaged cells. Then our body's helpful cells, like white blood cells, come to the site and help heal the damage. With COVID, there are multiple out-of-control areas that have harmful inflammation. The patient's immune system goes into overdrive, causing a cascade of potentially deadly effects, including lung failure, multiple blood clots, heart attack, and stroke.

How Coronavirus Affects the Different Organs in Our Body

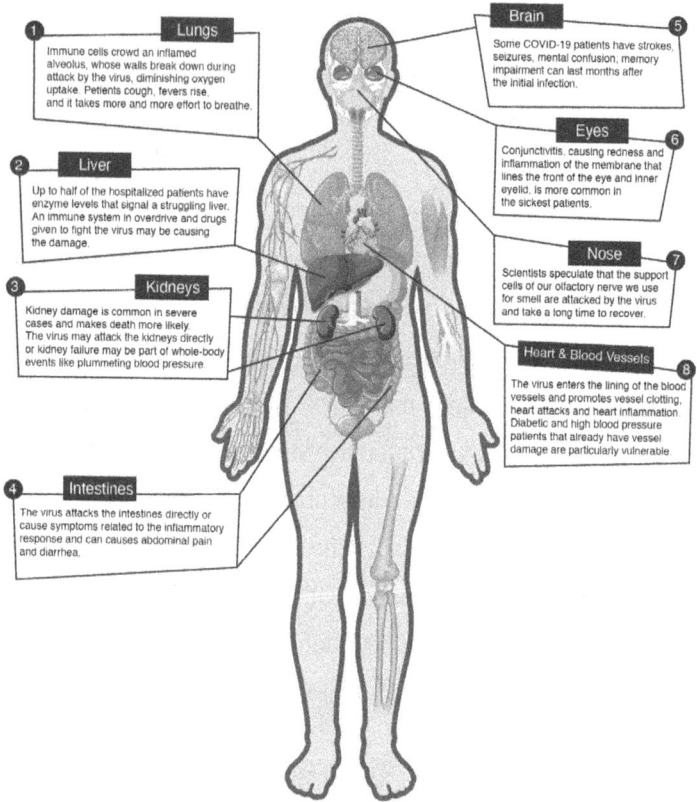

1 Lungs
Immune cells crowd an inflamed alveolus, whose walls break down during attack by the virus, diminishing oxygen uptake. Patients cough, fevers rise, and it takes more and more effort to breathe.

2 Liver
Up to half of the hospitalized patients have enzyme levels that signal a struggling liver. An immune system in overdrive and drugs given to fight the virus may be causing the damage.

3 Kidneys
Kidney damage is common in severe cases and makes death more likely. The virus may attack the kidneys directly or kidney failure may be part of whole-body events like plummeting blood pressure.

4 Intestines
The virus attacks the intestines directly or cause symptoms related to the inflammatory response and can causes abdominal pain and diarrhea.

5 Brain
Some COVID-19 patients have strokes, seizures, mental confusion, memory impairment can last months after the initial infection.

6 Eyes
Conjunctivitis, causing redness and inflammation of the membrane that lines the front of the eye and inner eyelid, is more common in the sickest patients.

7 Nose
Scientists speculate that the support cells of our olfactory nerve we use for smell are attacked by the virus and take a long time to recover.

8 Heart & Blood Vessels
The virus enters the lining of the blood vessels and promotes vessel clotting, heart attacks and heart inflammation. Diabetic and high blood pressure patients that already have vessel damage are particularly vulnerable.

The above image illustrates how COVID affects different organs. It is astounding how many organs the coronavirus can affect. The lung, kidney, and brain damage can last for months after the initial infection.

During the spring 2020 Chicago surge, my internal medicine, infectious disease, and pulmonary colleagues were constantly sharing information and tips on how to diagnose COVID. We quickly became familiar with the common COVID lung X-ray and computerized tomography (CT) findings. On both X-rays and chest CT scans, COVID-damaged lungs reveal a characteristic pattern, called "honeycombing" or "ground glass." The virus typically attacks the area between the alveoli and the blood vessels that exchange oxygen. A series of changes occurs in this area that decreases oxygen exchange. This results in the patient's oxygen level falling, sometimes dramatically. In later stages of the disease, there is an increased immune reaction, called a "cytokine storm," during which fluid collects in the lungs and alveoli. At this point, the patient is administered oxygen via a nasal cannula, an oxygen face mask, or a breathing machine or ventilator.

Increasingly, hospital rooms are equipped with higher-flow oxygen apparatuses in standard medical units. There is also a technique called "proning," in which the patient is placed in the prone (face down) position. This helps get oxygen to the part of the lungs that need it most.

COVID damages the blood vessels, which leads to increased clotting, especially in patients who are predisposed or who have already had vessel damage from diabetes and high blood pressure.

Clotting happens in our bodies regularly in a protective and organized way, but an increase in clotting in a disorganized way, which may occur with coronavirus, can be harmful. The body's reaction to the virus increases this aberrant clotting activity in a number of ways, including direct invasion of the blood vessels, which causes injury and an abnormal activation of the clotting system. The immune reaction is not limited to one part of the lungs, as in the case of bacterial pneumonia. Rather, this damaging immune reaction occurs throughout the entire lung and enters the bloodstream, affecting various organs including the liver, kidneys, heart, and brain.

Many of my COVID patients are curious as to how they lose their sense of taste and smell. The coronavirus attacks the supporting cells in the olfactory bulb of the nose, not the actual nerves we use to smell and taste. The supporting cells are rich in receptors that attract COVID. Our immune system replaces these supportive cells. This process of healing in the nose and returning to normal taste and smell can take a few weeks or even a couple of months.

As we can see, COVID can be destructive not only to the lungs, but also to many other parts of the body. No one really knows how it will interact with their system. Therefore, it's good to practice thorough COVID-preventive measures to keep yourself from getting the virus.

3 WHAT IS IMMUNITY?

"To lose patience is to lose the battle."
— Mahatma Gandhi

MANY OF MY PATIENTS DO not understand the concept of immunity or how it can protect them from getting COVID. In this chapter, I will explain immunity and clear up some of the myths.

Human beings have an elaborate and sophisticated immune system, which protects the body by fighting viruses, bacteria, and parasites. It "remembers" past invaders so that if one returns, it can be eliminated quickly by our body's elaborate system of defenses.

Vaccine immunity dependably results in a higher level of protective antibodies than we get with natural immunity—the immunity we develop by contracting COVID. We develop natural immunity as antibodies build up over three to four weeks following infection. The evidence to date suggests that natural immunity lasts for approximately six to eight months, and there are ongoing studies to confirm the duration of immunity following exposure.

There are three theories of how long vaccine immunity will last. The first theory is that COVID vaccine immunity will last about as long as natural immunity, which is six to eight months. The second theory is immunity will last about two years, and the third theory about five to ten years. Most immunologists believe that COVID vaccine immunity will last for about two years. The companies that make the vaccines are researching how long immunity will last and developing booster shots.

Of the two approved mRNA vaccines, the Pfizer-BioNTech vaccine, provides immunity as of seven days after the second dose, and the Moderna vaccine provides immunity fourteen days after the second dose.

Without vaccine immunity, individuals risk potentially irreversible damage to the body, and if one's immune system is not primed with a vaccine before exposure to the virus, the risk to the body is much greater. Our immune systems are extremely robust and can "remember" thousands of organisms and viruses and then attack the invaders, rendering them incapable of harming us.

Many of our routine childhood vaccinations are so effective that they provide lifelong immunity. Others need to be given periodically to maintain their effectiveness. We don't always know how an organism will affect the body–via the actual infection or from the body's immune response, which itself can be highly destructive. Hence, it's best to get immunized from potentially harmful infections as recommended by public health officials.

Young people often behave as though they're invincible, but they are actually at greater risk of overactive immune responses. Their bodies can become overwhelmed by the immune response, which can lead to death. Vaccines are mostly safe and are used worldwide, with a benefit-to-risk ratio that is probably greater than that of any other type of medical intervention. Vaccines will not keep infections from entering our bodies, but they can prevent viral loads from increasing to the point where the body might not even recognize that the infection is present. Most approved vaccines prevent serious disease and hospitalization, and this is a primary benefit of developing effective immunity to a particular pathogen.

4 HERD IMMUNITY

"In every crisis, doubt or confusion, take the higher path—the path of compassion, courage, understanding and love."

— Amit Ray

CONSIDERING THE ABOVE QUOTE IN regard to COVID, the path of compassion, courage, understanding, and love is getting the COVID vaccine and creating a herd immunity that protects all, including the most vulnerable in our society. In late spring 2021, at the time of this publication, there is a sense among some in the scientific community that herd immunity in the United States and the world may not be achievable. It has become apparent that many in our society are resistant to COVID vaccination. I believe we need to work harder to listen to individuals' doubts about the vaccine and yet push forward on a goal to attain COVID herd immunity.

I want normal! When are we going to have normal?! I am sure you want to get back to those magical days of 2019, when we could go to restaurants and movie theaters and meet in groups. But to do this, we need to understand what herd immunity is and how we get there. The sooner we get our population vaccinated, the sooner we can get back to a new normal. This new normal will not be the same as before, but we will be able do most of the things that we did before. We will still have to be vigilant—perhaps do a lot more handwashing and still wear masks under certain conditions, so the pandemic does not come back. I'm very optimistic that this new normal can be achieved and maintained if we all work together on the mitigation and we get vaccinated.

Granted, we're all going to have to participate in the mitigation process by masking, social distancing, and avoiding crowds for several more months. If we get enough of our population vaccinated, we can stop COVID in its tracks. Yes, it is actually possible—if we get 80 percent of our population vaccinated. The sooner we are all vaccinated, the sooner this pain and suffering can end.

Vaccine hesitancy, according to a World Health Organization (WHO) January 2019 report, was already a significant problem globally, resulting in three to four million people who could be saved if people weren't so hesitant about getting their vaccines when they are presented to them. Now with COVID, we have a greater opportunity to save lives by getting the vaccine as soon as possible. The sooner we get it, the more lives we will save. In other words, being on the fence about the vaccine has consequences. There are times in life to make a decision quickly, and this is one of those times.

So, let's explain this important concept of herd immunity in relation to COVID. Herd immunity occurs when a large enough portion of the population (known as the herd) collectively becomes immune to an infectious disease. This level of immunity (believed to be about 80 percent of the population in the case of COVID) stops the infection from spreading. Then, as a result, the entire community—whether a country or the entire global community—is shielded from the infection, not just those who are immune. In other words, COVID has nowhere to go and is stopped.

When herd immunity is reached, the vulnerable—the infants, the immunocompromised, and those with cancer, severe allergic reactions, or other conditions that prevent them from being vaccinated—will be protected.

In the early part of this pandemic, some countries thought to take the "natural immunity" approach—which is getting sick with COVID in order to acquire COVID antibodies, instead of the getting the vaccine. This practice didn't work well, because the antibodies did not last long, and the death rate of these countries was particularly high. Great Britain suggested they were going to do this during the early part of the of the epidemic, and perhaps many people did not participate in the robust precautionary mitigations. This lack of serious mitigations resulted in a higher infection rate and death rate in Great Britain for a period of time. Britain has since reversed its course, enacted stricter lockdowns, and has been very aggressive in its vaccination programs. Based on the available theories, it is believed that the vaccine immunity will likely last longer, perhaps one, two, or even ten years.

Once we achieve herd immunity from COVID, we need to follow public health guidelines in regard to when to get vaccinated again or when to get boosters to help protect us from COVID variants. The COVID vaccination process will not be a one-shot or two-shot series that results in lifelong immunity. Keeping up to date on your COVID vaccinations will likely be part of your future wellness regimen.

In other words, once we achieve herd immunity from COVID, we will actively have to maintain it. Measles in the United States had very high herd immunity as a result of an active national mass vaccination program, and by the year 2000, transmission was nearly zero. Since 2000, there have been a few years when measles started to come back because of vaccine hesitancy and low vaccination rates. For example, in 2019 there was a resurgence of measles in the United States. During that year, certain pockets of low herd immunity developed in the Pacific Northwest and in New York City particularly, and measles was a significant public health concern again.

How Herd Immunity Protects Us

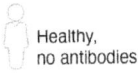

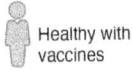

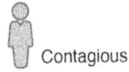

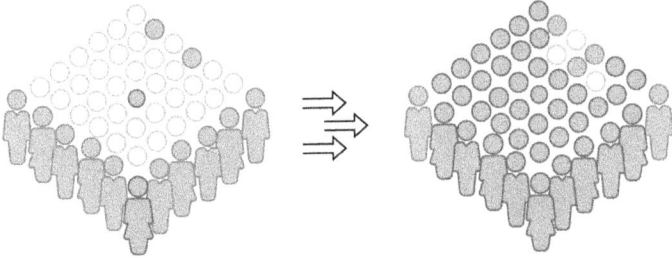

Healthy,
no antibodies

Healthy with
vaccines

Contagious

If only **some** have the antibodies or
have been vaccinated...

the virus easily **spreads**.

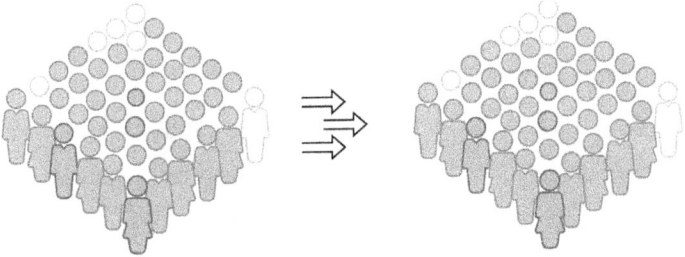

If **most** have the antibodies or
have been vaccinated...

the virus is **contained**.

The above diagram shows an excellent example of how herd immunity can stop COVID in its tracks.

The hollow blue dots and blue figures symbolize people that have not been vaccinated and are susceptible to getting COVID. The solid blue dots and solid blue figures symbolize those that were vaccinated. The red dots and red figures are those that contract COVID. These are two scenarios, and there is a time lapse from left to right. In the top scenario, not many are vaccinated. In the bottom scenario, several are vaccinated. So as time goes by, in the top scenario, of the people that are not vaccinated, about fifty get infected. This is what happens if COVID is left unchecked with few or no immune persons in a community. In the bottom scenario, over some time, the several vaccinated people, as illustrated by the solid blue dots and figures, block COVID from spreading. This may result in only one person getting infected, in essence stopping COVID in its tracks.

Vaccinated people literally act as human shields to protect those who cannot receive the vaccine because of allergic reactions or other medical conditions. The hope is that if we get 80 percent of the population vaccinated, along with those who have some natural immunity, coronavirus will absolutely decrease and maybe completely disappear.

If America achieves 50 percent herd immunity, we will have a much more protective effect than if no one got vaccinated. However, remember that, in that case, five out of ten of your herd could potentially give you coronavirus, instead of only two out of ten if 80 percent of the population was vaccinated. Achieving 50 percent herd immunity will be beneficial but will not be optimal. There will likely be fewer restrictions than before, but there will still be restrictions. So, let's all do our part, get vaccinated, and reach for 80 percent herd immunity, which will result in less suffering, death, and business closures and will allow our society to open up more freely. This 80 percent herd immunity for COVID is a good working percentage according to some experts at the time of this writing. The herd immunity percentage will always be a moving target. But for the purpose of this book, we will stick with the goal of 80 percent to bring the COVID transmission rate down enough to get back to a new normal.

Herd immunity depends on a number of factors, including how infectious COVID is, how effective the vaccine is (the Pfizer, Moderna, and Johnson & Johnson vaccines approved for emergency use to date are very effective), how long natural and vaccine immunity lasts, and how quickly everyone gets vaccinated. The variants, such as the predominant UK variant B.1.1.7, are 50 percent more infective than the common COVID. As the variants increase in the United States, infectivity increases, and the herd immunity percentage needed to stop COVID in its tracks goes up. So, to keep it simple, we need to make an impact and get as many in our communities vaccinated as possible in order to speed up herd immunity and decrease future mutations of COVID.

It is important to understand that if you have a highly infectious virus, it's much more important to attain a high level of herd immunity. See the example below of three viruses of varying infectivity.

To best understand how the coronavirus compares to other common viruses regarding herd immunity, we need to compare infectivity. With the yearly seasonal flu, one infected person infects about 1.3 people. With the coronavirus, one infected person infects approximately three people. With measles, one infected person infects about twelve people.

So, looking at the above infection rates, we can understand that the herd immunity percentage needs to be higher for more contagious illnesses like measles. The percentage of herd immunity needed for COVID is higher than the percentage for seasonal flu but lower than that for measles. Herd immunity for the seasonal flu is about 70 percent, herd immunity for COVID should be about 80 percent, and herd immunity for measles should be about 95 percent. We have attained and maintained a herd immunity over the last decade of over 90 percent for other contagious illnesses, so hopefully we can achieve the needed 80 percent herd immunity for COVID.

As I stated above, when considering vaccination and herd immunity, we also have to consider the efficacy of the vaccine. The first two vaccines approved in United States at 95 percent efficacy were Pfizer-BioNTech and Moderna. The Johnson & Johnson has about a 70 percent efficacy, so the average now is about 80 percent in United

States, and this 80 percent is probably going to stand. The higher the percentage of efficacy of the vaccine (or the more effective the vaccine), the fewer people that have to be vaccinated.

I believe we can reach herd immunity, because it has happened many times before during the last seventy years of vaccinations. Scores of organisms, bacterial and viral, have been successfully brought down by sustained vaccine programs over several years. There are three deadly viruses of note that have been brought under control by sustained mass vaccination programs. First, polio. During the height of the polio epidemic between 1950 and 1953, there were approximately 119,000 cases of paralytic polio and approximately 6,600 deaths in the United States. The US mass vaccination campaign started in 1955, and by 1979 there were no cases of polio that had originated in the United States.

Second, smallpox was wiped off the face of the earth by a successful vaccination program. The smallpox virus has likely been on earth since 10,000 BC. Scientists have found evidence of smallpox lesions in some of the 3,000-year-old mummies in Egypt. It is estimated that smallpox may have killed 300 to 500 million people in the twentieth century alone. WHO started a smallpox mass eradication program in 1966, and by 1980 this deadly virus had been eradicated from the world.

Finally, measles was the number one cause of death in children in the United States during the first half of the twentieth century.

Throughout the 1960s, about 400 to 500 people per year died of measles in the United States. In 1979, the Centers for Disease Control (CDC) started a mass vaccination campaign against measles, and by 1982 the measles infection rate had dropped by 80 percent. By the year 2000, measles was effectively wiped out in the United States.

Because of vaccine hesitancy since the year 2000, there's been a measles outbreak, which was especially significant in 2019 in certain pockets in the US—namely, the Pacific Northwest and New York. So these three examples of mass vaccination against deadly viruses gives me confidence that if we have a sustained COVID vaccine program we can attain the same protective herd immunity and stop COVID in its tracks.

The final takeaway message of this chapter is that if you and your herd do your part, we can end this pandemic and get back to near normal life. The phrase "think globally, act locally" has been used in various contexts to encourage us to do our part in our communities. The phrase urges us to consider the health of the entire planet. We do this by taking action in our own backyard, our community of family, friends, and coworkers.

We hear these big, scary concepts in regard to the pandemic on the news, but let us not be deterred by bad news. We have to determine what we need to do in our part of the world to make it better. Educate, encourage, convince, or cajole your small herd of ten people to do masking and hand sanitizing, and encourage everybody to get the COVID vaccine. Focus on stopping COVID within your own small herd. If millions of small herds across the country are successful too, we will achieve a new normal.

5 UNDERSTANDING VACCINES

"In the face of adversity, we have a choice: we can be bitter or we can be better."

— Caryn Sullivan

AT THE TIME OF THIS writing, the three approved vaccines for COVID are from Pfizer-BioNTech, Moderna, and Johnson & Johnson. According to the CDC, all three vaccines have similar common side effects, including injection-site pain, redness, and swelling. Other side effects include tiredness, headache, muscle pain, chills, fever, and nausea. Severe allergic reactions, or anaphylaxis, occur in approximately 1 in 100,000 cases, and nearly always within the first fifteen minutes. All vaccine centers have a monitoring period of at least fifteen to thirty minutes after giving the vaccine. The rate of allergic reactions to the COVID vaccine is ten times greater than that for the flu shot, which is 1 in 1 million, but they are rare and treatable reactions.

Allergic reactions to COVID vaccines are usually caused by lipids, electrolytes, and preservatives in the vaccine. If a patient has had a previous severe allergic reaction to a vaccine ingredient, that patient should not get the COVID vaccine. If a patient has a severe allergic reaction to the first shot, then they should not have the second shot.

STAGGERING IMPROVEMENT IN QUALITY OF LIFE AS A RESULT OF VACCINES OVER THE PAST TWO CENTURIES

To fully appreciate how vaccines have advanced public health, it is useful to reflect on how far we've come in the 230 years since the advent of modern vaccinations. If not for vaccines, we would have rampant illness in our society, including horrific rashes on our arms and legs, physical deformities, and paralysis. These conditions are still present in third-world countries in varying degrees. Everyone benefits from the improved health and the increased average longevity that vaccines have brought.

Mass vaccination programs are not new; we simply haven't had one for several decades. Hence, we have been lulled into a false sense of security that we no longer need to worry about infectious disease outbreaks. However, as COVID has amply demonstrated, we are still vulnerable to previously unknown infectious disease agents.

DEBUNKING MEDICAL MYTHS ABOUT COVID VACCINES

Many people fear vaccines. I would like to help allay those fears by addressing some of the common myths about the COVID vaccine:

1. "If I've already had COVID, I don't need a vaccine."

    FALSE.

    Those who were asymptomatic and had a mild infection usually don't have strong enough immune protection. Those who have had moderate or severe COVID may have some protection, but we're not certain for how long they will have protective antibodies. The vaccine provides a more dependable and robust protection with a high degree of immunity.

2. "You can get COVID from the COVID vaccine."

    FALSE.

    Just as it is impossible to get the flu from the flu shot, it's impossible to get COVID from the COVID vaccine. All approved vaccines have safe forms of either deactivated virus or small components of the virus.

3. "Some COVID vaccines enter your cells and change your DNA."

FALSE.

Current approved vaccines use the mRNA. This is a different genetic message than DNA. The mRNA goes into the cell's ribosomes, that is, the "protein factories" within our cells that produce proteins. It never enters the nucleus and so cannot be incorporated into DNA. Moreover, the mRNA introduced by the vaccine is discarded after a brief period, but the harmless proteins remain. These proteins produce antibodies that provide the protective immunity.

4. "The COVID vaccine can affect women's fertility."

FALSE.

An unfortunate false report from social media claimed that the spike protein used in the two approved vaccines is similar to a protein that is used in the attachment of the placenta during pregnancy. In fact, the proteins are not similar, and COVID vaccines have no impact on fertility.

It is my hope that this chapter has given you some more information so you can make an informed decision regarding vaccines. We have had a pandemic thrust upon us suddenly and have to make timely decisions about vaccines for our loved ones. I recommend that everyone learn about and understand the importance of vaccines in our lives. By focusing on credible medical sources, you will find answers to your questions about the COVID vaccines. It is my hope that this book and its references will help you in your decision-making process.

6 THE VACCINE DEVELOPMENT PROCESS AND COVID VACCINES

"Life doesn't get easier or more forgiving; we get stronger and more resilient."

– Steve Maraboli

AN IMPORTANT CONSIDERATION DURING AN epidemic or pandemic is the sequencing of the virus. We need to understand the virus in order to understand what antivirals will be effective in treating it and what vaccine strategies will be effective in defeating it.

Today there are some two hundred COVID vaccines in devolvement or developed. The *New York Times* has an extensive database, the "Coronavirus Vaccine Tracker," that is very helpful and describes the progress of the vaccines and how each of them works.

PHASES OF VACCINE DEVELOPMENT

Preclinical testing – The "pre" part means before human testing. The first tests are "in vitro," meaning they are conducted on cells, and that is followed by "in vivo" tests, those conducted on living animals such as mice or monkeys. Vaccine candidates are tested to determine whether they will elicit an immune response. If not, then the vaccine candidate does not go on to phase 1 human studies. Scientists may test existing vaccine techniques or totally new techniques. If they discover an effective vaccine technique that produces a protective immune reaction, then the research proceeds to phase 1.

Phase 1 – In this phase, scientists administer the vaccine candidate to a small number of healthy volunteers, usually between twenty and eighty, to determine whether it is safe and whether the immune response works in people. To determine if it's safe, they observe symptoms for seven days after each vaccination, The primary focus is on safety, but this phase is also used to gain preliminary or for as much as a month. evidence that the medication is effective against the disease or condition. If phase 1 is successful, then the vaccine candidate moves on to phase 2 testing.

Phase 2 – During phase 2, test subjects are divided in two groups; one group receives the vaccine and the other receives a placebo. Subjects of these groups usually number in the hundreds. This phase further tests the vaccine's safety. The side effects are evaluated in this phase.

Phase 3 – The study continues with placebo and vaccine groups consisting of thousands of individuals per group, which helps determine the vaccine's effectiveness. In the case of the Pfizer-BioNTech and Moderna vaccines, their efficacy rate in phase 3 trials was 95 percent. The threshold to be approved is 50 percent effectiveness, so 95 percent is astounding. Further data showed that both of these vaccines give people a nearly 100 percent chance of not being hospitalized.

Emergency or limited approval – This is a designation given by certain countries in approving vaccines to be administered to certain groups. In the United States, this is called emergency use authorization (EUA). The Food and Drug Administration (FDA) is the body that issues EUAs. In the case of both the Pfizer-BioNTech and Moderna vaccines, the US CDC also gave full approval shortly after the FDA allowed EUA. Some countries, such as China and Russia, do not wait for the results of phase 3 trials before giving vaccines early approval.

Full approval – After regular review of complete trial results, the regulatory body of the country approves the vaccine. In the US, the regulatory body is the FDA.

Major strategies of vaccine development

GENETIC-CODE VACCINES
Pfizer / BioNTech, Moderna

Selective viral DNA or RNA fragments elicit an immune response

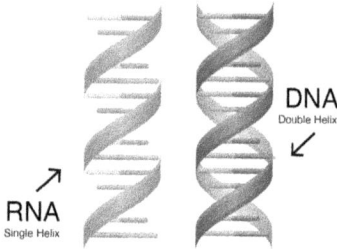

RNA
Single Helix

DNA
Double Helix

VIRAL VECTOR VACCINES
AstraZeneca/Oxford, J&J, Cansino

Selective DNA and RNA fragments placed in a more sturdy shell elicit an immune response

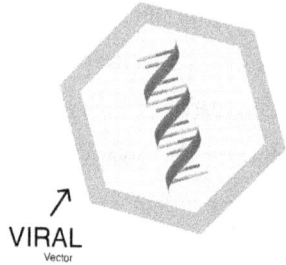

VIRAL
Vector

SUBUNIT VACCINES`
Novavax

Parts of the infective organism as proteins elicit an immune response

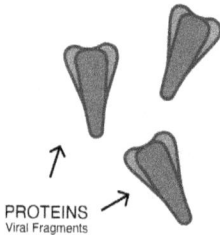

PROTEINS
Viral Fragments

WEAKENED / INACTIVE VACCINES
Sinovac, Sinopharm

Inactivated or dead infective organisms elicit an immune response

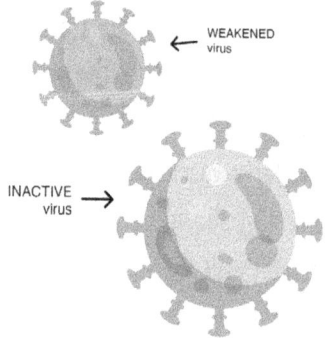

WEAKENED
virus

INACTIVE
virus

The above picture illustrates the four major global COVID vaccine strategies.

In the next section, I will lay out the four major vaccines' mechanisms of action and give a brief description of each one that is being used in the United States.

MRNA VACCINES

Pfizer-BioNTech and Moderna both use this technology to develop this type of vaccine, and so we'll discuss these two vaccines together. Pfizer developed a vaccine called tozinameran, under the brand name Comirnaty, and Moderna's vaccine is called mRNA-1273.

In chapter 1, the "Anatomy of the Coronavirus" section showed that the outside of the coronavirus has spike proteins that attach to receptors in our body's cells to infect them. The code for making proteins is mRNA. Both the Pfizer and Moderna vaccines have a form of mRNA. This mRNA sequence is the code for the outer spike protein. The viral mRNA sequence enters our cells and uses the ribosomes to create proteins that make only the spikes, not the entire virus. Remember from chapter 1 that there are about one hundred spikes that project out from an intact coronavirus. The spikes themselves do not cause disease, but they do cause the immune system to recognize the coronavirus and produce antibodies. Hence, should the actual coronavirus appear, the body's immune system will recognize and quickly destroy it.

In the case of the Pfizer-BioNTech vaccine, the fragile mRNA is encased in an oily bubble. The bubbles bump into our cells, and the coded mRNA builds the spike proteins. We don't need to worry about this strip of mRNA being coded into our DNA; the mRNA is destroyed, leaving no trace of any genetic material.

Through a series of steps, antibodies are created that recognize spike proteins as foreign invaders. The antibodies destroy the coronavirus in a couple of ways. First, they identify and attack the spike protein part of the coronavirus before the virus can enter our body's cells. The antibodies also send signals to recruit other cells, such as killer T cells, that destroy the virus directly.

COMPARING THE TWO MRNA VACCINES, PFIZER-BIONTECH AND MODERNA

There are slight differences in the ingredients of the two vaccines. The major difference is that the Pfizer vaccine has to be stored at very low temperatures (-94°F), whereas the Moderna vaccine can be shipped and stored at less cold temperatures (-4°F). The Pfizer vaccine is approved for administration to individuals sixteen years old and up, and the Moderna vaccine is for those eighteen years old and up. The ingredients, listed below, are similar, with some proprietary differences. Both Pfizer-BioNTech and Moderna are two-dose vaccines. The two Pfizer doses are administered three weeks apart and the Moderna doses are administered four weeks apart.

The two lists below show the ingredients of both the Pfizer-BioNTech and the Moderna vaccines. Notice that the lists are very similar. These lists are relevant because those with severe allergic reactions are usually allergic to one or more of the components in the vaccine that is used as a preservative.

Pfizer-BioNTech

mRNA

Lipids

Potassium chloride

Monobasic potassium phosphate

Sodium chloride

Dibasic sodium phosphate dihydrate

Sucrose

Moderna

mRNA

Lipids

Tromethamine

Tromethamine hydrochloride

Acidic acid

Sodium acetate

Sucrose

VIRAL VECTOR VACCINES

This class of vaccines uses a virus shell that carries coronavirus genes. Oxford-AstraZeneca and Johnson & Johnson have developed viral vector vaccines. First, a modified version of an adenovirus, a more benign type of virus, is developed. Then the coronavirus DNA is placed inside this modified adenovirus shell, as shown in the above illustration. The advantage of this viral vector vaccine is that it is a more robust way of encapsulating genetic material than the fragile oil bubbles that the mRNA vaccines use. The greatest advantage of this is that the vaccine can last for at least six months when refrigerated in a standard refrigerator at 38–46°F. Hence, this vaccine can be more effective globally, especially in areas where the infrastructure to maintain the extreme refrigeration temperatures required by the other vaccines is not available.

The DNA particle encased in the modified adenovirus enters the vaccinated cell. Once inside the cell, the DNA is injected into the nucleus and then converted to mRNA. The mRNA goes outside the nucleus of the cell, and the same process occurs as with an mRNA vaccine to achieve immunity. The Ebola vaccine uses this technology as well.

PROTEIN-BASED AND SUBUNIT VACCINES

Novavax uses this protein-based technology, which creates a nanoparticle with multiple spike proteins that band to each other. These nanoparticles are created in a lab before they are injected. Scientists insert the gene that codes for the DNA of the spike protein into the DNA of baculovirus. The result is production of the spike proteins, banded together. These nanoparticles, along with immunity priming compounds, are injected into the patient. This initiates the same immune process that occurs after the spike proteins are formed in all of the methods described above.

Sanofi and GlaxoSmithKline both use similar protein-based technologies for their vaccines.

INACTIVATED OR ATTENUATED VACCINES

This technique is used for many different types of existing vaccines. The virus is first made inactive, or killed, or attenuated. The incapacitated virus will not make you sick but will elicit an immune response. Inactivated or attenuated coronavirus vaccines have been developed by China, India, and Russia, and there are also other vaccine techniques being used.

I believe that from this flurry of vaccine development we will learn vital techniques to help us face future epidemics and pandemics. I also believe that we will develop additional booster vaccines and other vaccines that will be more effective against new variants of coronavirus and other viruses in the future.

7 19 REASONS TO GET THE COVID-19 VACCINATION

DURING MOST IN-PERSON OFFICE OR telemedicine visits, I discuss the COVID vaccine as the best way for COVID prevention. Many of my patients say things like, "Doctor, it's been so hard, and I'm just overwhelmed in dealing with COVID. Thank you, but really, it's just too much. I don't know if I can talk about vaccines right now." My patients' initial overwhelming feeling dissipated after a few weeks, when I gave them more information about how the vaccine was a way out of the restricted lifestyles we've all been living for so many months.

I certainly understand that COVID is an overwhelming challenge to deal with day to day. I had the advantage of studying the virus extensively with several MDs who conducted clinical and research clerkships under my supervision. My medical team and I developed the confidence to counsel my patients and present them with a viable pathway toward normalcy. I came to an understanding of and peace with COVID and found ways to beat the virus.

At the time of this publication, in the United States there are three vaccines approved for emergency use authorization (EUA), and millions of Americans are receiving them. All three of these vaccines remain in phase 3 and have not gotten FDA approval. As time goes by and we vaccinate the public, we are discovering added benefits of these vaccines, like that they have activity against the newly discovered COVID variants like the UK variant, B.1.17 and the Indian variant, Delta Plus. We also may uncover potential risks of the vaccines. Each time a side effect occurs after vaccine administration, we have to look at it scientifically and try to understand exactly what happened. Scientists carefully determine if the side effect occurred coincidentally or was related to the vaccine. Then they consider other ways to administer the vaccine to potentially prevent the side effect. Analyzing a new vaccine side effect is a rigorous process that takes time, and we must be patient to wait for the final recommendations.

As with any medical issue, I had to calm my patients' acute concerns first—in this case, their overall fear of COVID. Then, over a period of weeks and several visits, I was able to talk about the vaccine. Because I knew it would be a hard sell in our vaccine-hesitant society, I started talking about COVID vaccines well before any of the vaccines were approved in the United States in August 2020. I would include this discussion in every patient encounter. After hundreds of these conversations over a period of several months, I gained a deep understanding of the many questions, concerns, and fears about the vaccines. From those conversations, I developed arguments for convincing patients that the COVID vaccine is the best way to return to normal life.

I would often point out that the two words "COVID" and "vaccine" elicit fear. It is perfectly rational to be afraid of COVID; if you're not afraid of it, you're not looking at reality. However, the fear generated by the second word, "vaccine," is not rational. It stems from twenty years of medical misinformation. People are logically afraid of COVID, but illogically afraid of vaccines. I will discuss the truth about vaccines in much greater detail in this chapter. Vaccines are, in general, safe and effective, and they have very few side effects.

Below are 19 reasons to get the COVID-19 vaccine. I actually came up with many more reasons, but I decided these were the most important to me and they're the ones that came up quite often in discussion with my patients. Also, it was a bit poetic to provide 19 reasons to get the COVID-19 vaccine.

1. **You can save your own life and the lives of hundreds of thousands**

By getting the vaccine, you're not only protecting yourself from COVID, but you are also bringing humanity one step closer to ending the virus's ability to harm us. If enough people in your community are vaccinated, then your community will have protective herd immunity. You have slowed the virus to a trickle and will eventually stop it in its tracks. Just imagine for a moment that we had no vaccine at all. This would be a very sad scenario. It is estimated that if we had not had a vaccine beginning in December 2020, an extra 900,000 Americans would have died. Luckily, this is not our fate. At the time of this writing, 45 percent of Americans have already been fully vaccinated. I received both doses of the Pfizer vaccine without incident, by mid-January 2021. It is important to get the full recommended regimen of the vaccine; the Johnson & Johnson vaccine is one shot, and Pfizer and Moderna are two-shot regimens.

By getting vaccinated, you can help save thousands of lives, and our health care system can go back to treating patients suffering from other illnesses. Many patients have not received adequate treatment due to hospitals being overwhelmed with COVID patients. Hospitals can only treat so many patients, and COVID has stretched their capacity to the limit. We need our hospitals for heart attacks, strokes, and trauma. At present, the health care system has much more limited capacity to accommodate other urgent medical issues. The US will undoubtedly recover from COVID, but some countries' health care systems have been devastated and they will need help rebuilding their fragile health care resources once the pandemic is over.

The average cost of caring for a COVID patient is between $20,000 and $80,000. Therefore, every individual who is vaccinated potentially decreases the burden on our health care system, allowing hospitals to recover so that people can receive the treatments they need for other serious health issues. Millions of Americans have already been vaccinated, and we are making steady progress. Please do your part.

2. **Vaccination will protect you from COVID-19**

The COVID vaccines that have been approved, in United States and globally, have shown very impressive results, not only in preventing COVID but also in preventing large numbers of people from needing hospitalization. For many people, vaccination prevents coronavirus from reproducing significantly in our bodies hence, it is likely that it will decrease transmission significantly. After vaccination, it is still possible to have upper respiratory symptoms such as a cough and sore throat, but the vaccine will protect you from the worst symptoms, including pneumonia and other illnesses caused or exacerbated by COVID.

It should be mentioned that the coronavirus can still enter your body, but you may not even realize it. One or two weeks after you receive your COVID vaccine, your immune system will be completely ready to protect you from the virus.

3. **Current COVID-19 vaccines are safe**

Vaccine development is an extremely rigorous process, and the safety profiles of the overwhelming majority of vaccines are excellent. In general, and with the COVID vaccine in particular, approximately one in every 100,000 individuals will experience a serious reaction to the vaccine, usually an allergic reaction. Most allergic reactions occur within thirty minutes of the injection, and so monitoring recipients is a simple matter of observing them post-injection. If a reaction does occur, the patient can seek treatment quickly and safely. I have administered hundreds of flu shots in my medical office over the past six years and have never seen a single allergic reaction. I myself have had flu shots every year for the past twenty years and have never had an allergic reaction.

Other common side effects from the injection include muscle soreness, swelling, body aches, headache, fever, and weakness.

The COVID vaccines that have been approved so far have the same 1-in-100,000 odds of severe allergic reaction as vaccines in general. The side effects of COVID vaccines are also similar; some people have more significant side effects after the second COVID shot, but these symptoms are short-lived, most lasting a couple of days or sometimes a week.

4. Current COVID vaccines are highly effective

The average efficacy of the flu shot is about 50 percent, which means that it will prevent the flu about 50 percent of the time. This is a different process, as flu shots are meant to protect us from several different influenza viruses. The COVID vaccine is for one virus only. The efficacy of the AstraZeneca vaccine is about 70 percent. It is estimated that the average efficacy of all the COVID vaccines is 80 percent, which is a tremendous achievement. It means that, on average, those who get the vaccine will be protected from COVID about 80 percent of the time.

At the end of 2020, I was curious as to the efficacy of the vaccines under development. Along with the rest of the health care community, I was absolutely amazed when I heard that both the Pfizer-BioNTech and the Moderna vaccine had efficacy rates of 95 percent. The goal for all of the programs in the US was to achieve an efficacy rate greater than 50 percent. The first three vaccines approved for emergency use far surpassed that 50 percent bar.

5. The benefits of COVID vaccination strongly outweigh the risks

Your risk of getting COVID, having long-term complications, or dying are much greater than any of the potential risks–including allergic reactions and other side effects–of the currently approved vaccines. In comparison, antibiotics, which are used routinely to treat a wide variety of infections, including pneumonia, meningitis, and blood infections, have a far greater potential for side effects than vaccines, including a high frequency of severe allergic reaction, rashes, diarrhea, low blood pressure, and weakness. Yet most of us take antibiotics, despite the truth that they have worse side effects. We should better balance benefit and risk, and the risk of having a side effect with the COVID vaccine is a lot less than with most medicines.

6. **No shortcuts were taken in the development of the currently approved vaccines**

Many people I have spoken with are concerned about the speed at which the vaccines were created, tested, and brought to market.

Public health officials were prudent in the spring of 2020, when it became apparent that COVID was going to be a serious global health problem. They stated that, even at an accelerated pace, it would take a year to a year and a half to develop a vaccine. Normally, vaccines take five to ten years to develop.

I reviewed the timeline, key research, and impressive data from Pfizer-BioNTech and Moderna. All of the steps in vaccine development were there. Even though development took just ten months, no corners were cut. I had my first Pfizer vaccine injection on Friday, December 18, 2020–at the end of the first week the vaccine became available in the United States. I was euphoric and had a sense of peace when I got my second dose in January 2021.

In reviewing the vaccine development data, I came to understand why the COVID vaccines were developed at a much faster rate. First, six US companies received billions of dollars in funding immediately, which is a process that usually takes many months or even years. Second, many techniques have been developed, such as PCR, to speed the process along. Third, unlike most vaccine development initiatives, which are typically done independently by individual pharmaceutical companies, there has been immense sharing of information worldwide. During the first few months of development, all six vaccine companies committed to total transparency with their data. Even the article publication process was sped up if it was related to vaccine development. Fourth, phases 2 and 3, the safety and efficacy steps, were combined, saving valuable time. Fifth, the FDA expedited the approval process. Finally, the scientists worked night and day due to the urgency of the situation. The process was the fastest of its kind in history, but in the end, no steps were skipped.

7. To prevent exposure to COVID-19's unknown potential long-term effects

More time and research are needed before we will fully understand all the long-term impacts of COVID. I have read in the literature and seen for myself in my COVID hospital patients some of the more common long-term complications, including lung manifestations, various blood-clotting problems, and kidney damage.

COVID damages the body in a number of ways. The coronavirus enters several organs, resulting in damage from both the virus itself and the body's strong and widespread immune reaction. These long-term complications are covered in greater detail in chapter 2.

8. **To protect your loved ones from contracting COVID**

The best way to protect loved ones is by being vaccinated. This creates a little cocoon of love and immunity to COVID. The people we care about need to get vaccinated to protect not only themselves but others close to them. This is a way of creating herd immunity on a small scale.

Herd immunity is an extremely important concept regarding infectious diseases. I define and discuss herd immunity in greater detail in chapter 4. As a brief reminder, herd immunity refers to achieving a critical level of immunity across a given population by vaccinating enough individuals to slow the spread of the virus to the point that it can be managed safely and effectively.

The clear advantage of nearly everyone in your household or other close group being vaccinated is that you will create an "immunity bubble," thereby significantly decreasing the risk of infection for those in your group who are not vaccinated.

Start initiating discussions with those who are close to you. Emphasize that taking a "wait and see" approach is a dangerous choice. As mentioned in other parts of the book, coronavirus will not stop until 60–70 percent of the population has been vaccinated. Even if you've had COVID once, you can get it again, and those close to you can also get it again. There is great benefit in being vaccinated, to you and your "herd" of about ten people with whom you associate regularly, including household members, family, close friends, coworkers, and neighbors.

If you stay within your bubble of ten mostly vaccinated people, your chances of contracting COVID when you venture outside your bubble to go to the grocery store or run other errands are extremely low. You will have created an immunity zone among your small herd. Then, if someone infected with COVID comes into contact with you or others in your group, your group's robust vaccine immunity will protect you. In essence, your group will have created a "big immunity shield" against COVID. Moreover, you and your group members won't infect other small herds. In time, the numbers will fall to the point where we can return to normal life.

9. To effectively, quickly, and safely achieve global herd immunity

On average, the currently approved COVID vaccines have an efficacy rate of about 80 percent. So as more people get the vaccine, the transmission rate continues to decrease. Vaccination is the only effective way to achieve protective herd immunity. Simply put, it is a cure for the pandemic. It is the only realistic pathway to a near-normal, post-pandemic world. There is not any other way to achieve this. It's been discussed by experts that if the pandemic is not controlled and contained quickly, there's a greater likelihood that it will go on for much longer, especially with new variants occurring. Mass vaccination is also the best way to prevent new variants.

10. **To achieve herd immunity with compassion for others.**

I grew up in a big, gregarious Italian family, and I learned early on to be respectful to those of other races, ethnicities, and religions. This foundation has given me a fulfilling life. Learning how my patients see the world continues to enrich my life and give it more meaning. When I go to television conferences to pitch my health show, I call myself, "Kumbaya guy," a people person. When I say this, others warm up to me and we have a good networking session.

Social media (and spending more time in front of screens in general, along with other lifestyle factors) has made us more isolated and less connected to our communities than ever before. Since moving to Chicago a number of years ago, I've seen people keeping more to themselves and reaching out to strangers less often. We need to be less isolated and reach out to neighbors, and even strangers. I'm trying to sell you on being a "Kumbaya" person. Make an effort to care about your fellow human beings and connect in a real, human way. Doing so will benefit you in your life in general, and it will help end this pandemic sooner. We need to work together with compassion to make it happen.

Try venturing beyond your comfort zone. Reach out to those who are vulnerable and might not understand the importance of wearing masks, social distancing, and getting vaccinated. It's true that those who contract COVID and survive may provide some degree of immunity, but many will suffer and die, and this is not a humane way to achieve herd immunity. The safest, most effective way to achieve herd immunity is for as many of us as possible to get vaccinated and convince those around us—even strangers we meet—to do so as well.

11. **Vaccination is the fastest route back to normalcy**

As mentioned in reason 9, the COVID vaccines are the quickest, most effective way to achieve herd immunity, and herd immunity is essential to returning to normal life. Achieving herd immunity is perhaps the most immediate goal, but there are other elements needed to enhance public safety. We need to have reliable sources of public health information, including traditional news media, websites, and discerning, well-informed individuals. It's important to stay well informed as pandemic conditions change and improve.

If you don't have a primary care doctor, now would be a good time to get one. Your doctor can provide valuable advice for your COVID-preventive health, along with other important measures for staying healthy, vigilant, and safe.

It is believed that COVID vaccine boosters, including those for new COVID variants, may come out from time to time. It's important to understand this and to actively seek out the recommended booster shots to keep yourself safe, as well as those around you. I believe that if we do all of these things, we can safely return to normal life, including dining out at restaurants, attending social gatherings, going to concerts, and–my personal favorite–going to the movies.

12. **To free up hospital and health-care resources used to fight COVID-19**

We've all heard stories on the news during COVID surges, from New York City to the Dakotas, related to limited hospital beds, critical care resources, intensive care personnel, ventilators and other equipment, PPE, and other essential hospital supplies. Sadly, there have been situations in which hospitals simply did not have enough intensive care rooms or ventilators, and doctors had to make difficult decisions as to which patients should get these scarce resources, resulting in others dying.

During the Chicago COVID surge in April 2020, I had to call four hospitals to find an intensive care unit (ICU) bed. I had a patient in the emergency room of one of the hospitals. Fortunately, I was on staff at several hospitals, and I was able to get that patient an ICU bed.

Working in hospitals for the past twenty years, I have seen that hospitals under stress are less effective in caring for patients. Mass vaccinations will bring down COVID numbers and allow not only more efficient allocation of resources, but also reduce the stress that ultimately hurts all patients.

13. **To help the economy return to normal and help the millions who lost their jobs return to work**

The retail, local transportation, travel, and hospitality sectors have been hit hardest by the COVID pandemic. The unemployment rate in leisure and hospitality went from 5 percent in late 2019 to 16.7 percent one year later. Unemployment in the construction industry nearly doubled, from 5 percent to 9.6 percent, during the same period. The motion picture industry unemployment rate tripled, from about 2 percent to 6.4 percent. The unemployment rate for self-employed individuals more than doubled, from 2.7 percent to 6.7 percent by the end of 2020.

Small businesses are particularly vulnerable to the sort of disruption that we are experiencing now, given that they lack the cash reserves to survive prolonged loss of business. Revenue losses resulted not only from the government shutting down businesses, but also from decreased demand by customers who did not venture out of their homes unless it was absolutely necessary. This resulted in severe revenue losses for restaurants, hotels, retail stores, and movie theaters. Returning to normal life will likely take several months as consumer confidence slowly returns, even after COVID cases are under control.

Interrupting this vicious downward economic cycle requires that we limit COVID cases in our communities, and the best way to achieve this is to get the vaccine.

14. **To stop living in fear**

Our COVID fears, whether founded or unfounded, can bring us down to the point that we can be paralyzed. Just like any fear or stress, we have to bring it out in the open by discussing it with a friend or a professional.

I included more advice on these concerns in chapter 8. Here, I'll relate some of the common stress factors that my patients have. First, they fear that they have COVID, even though their symptoms are not consistent with COVID. Second, they're confused and stressed out about their COVID test results. Third, they're anxious about the pandemic and don't know when it's going to be over. Fourth, when a patient contracts COVID, they fear worse outcomes than are justified by the severity of their symptoms. Finally, after a patient's COVID is resolved, they often experience weakness for a short period, which is partly related to COVID, but it also stems from their obsessive anxiety.

All of these fears can be addressed. Make sure you tell your doctor or a trusted support person about how you are feeling and work through these feelings logically, supported with sound public health data from sites such as cdc.org. Some of my patients who already have mental health and anxiety issues have been nearly paralyzed with fear of the virus. I do my best to help them let go of their stress. Don't bottle up or hide your COVID stress and fears; seek out a primary care doctor and a support person who is honest and can talk to you about your COVID concerns.

I myself experienced a significant increase in stress. When the pandemic began, I was fearful when the Chicago surge came, from March through May 2020. I have always counseled my patients on stress management, and I thought I had good coping skills. However, during the spring Chicago surge, I had a hard time adjusting. I was very stressed out at times, and I adjusted not only my day-to-day life, but also my professional life. Moreover, I had to learn how to use additional personal protective equipment (PPE) correctly. I remember sitting in the parking lot outside St. Mary's hospital, watching PPE videos before going inside to see my first COVID patient. The videos were made during the Ebola epidemic and demonstrated how to use PPE. On the previous day, I was "fit tested" by a nurse to ensure that there was a tight seal with my PPE, and to make sure I was wearing my shield and that everything was functioning properly before I saw any COVID patients.

A few months earlier, I had heard stories of some Italian doctors who had not used their PPE correctly. They were exposed, and they contracted COVID and died. I was terrified while walking in to see my first COVID patient. It took me about three months and extensive research with my colleagues to feel comfortable with PPE and seeing COVID patients.

When you're overwhelmed with fear, reach out to a medical professional who has a strong grasp of COVID information and who can listen empathetically.

15. **To help those who have suffered work and school disruptions to return to their normal life**

Containing the virus requires that we all develop new habits, including masking, shielding, and social distancing. Some of these protocols can be tedious and difficult while we're working or going to school. Unfortunately, there's no way around this, and the sooner we accept the new reality, the easier it will be to make it part of our everyday lives. The process will take some time, and we need to be patient, but it will get easier once it becomes part of our daily routines.

All of the mitigation processes put in place by federal, state, and local governments and by companies and schools will become less necessary over time. Furthermore, every additional person vaccinated will help them go away sooner. As we near the 80 percent vaccination level goal, we'll move closer to normal life. Once we reach 30 percent immunity, perhaps most schools and colleges can safely reopen for in-person learning. When we achieve 40 or 50 percent immunity, restrictions will be lifted on restaurants and retail stores. Every additional vaccinated person gets us closer.

16. **To stop the COVID-19 virus from mutating**

People are somewhat concerned about mutations of the virus, and it's useful to put this in perspective. There is still a very high risk of contracting the original COVID, and reducing this risk to those of herd immunity levels is still very much our primary goal. The drug companies are working on new vaccines for treating the variants. At the time of this publication, there are three existing worrisome international variants: the UK variant, the South African variant, and the Brazilian variant. Most of the existing variants–the three international variants and some other domestic ones–are likely to be prevented by the currently approved vaccines. Moreover, mutations occur when there are very large numbers of infected individuals (millions, as there are now) and so getting vaccinated will help prevent future mutations.

At the time of this writing, there are six known variants, three of which are of greater concern. The six variants include the UK, South African, Brazilian, California, New York, and Ohio variants. The first ones, originating in other countries beginning in fall 2020, are the most significant. More studies are being conducted on the existing variants across the United States, but so far, the UK, South African, and Brazilian variants are more dangerous, and so I will focus on them. In late February 2021, the FDA established guidelines on how to manage current and future variants.

The UK variant was identified in the US in December 2020. This variant is about 50 percent more infective than common COVID, and it has now spread to every state. At the time of this writing, the UK variant is the dominant strain in the US, and it is believed to be more deadly than common COVID. A study conducted in Britain noted the increased fatality rate. More studies need to be conducted to confirm the findings. Researchers believe that all of the vaccines currently approved in the United States are effective against this variant.

The South African variant, first detected in late January 2021, is the second most common variant active in the US. At the time of this writing (spring 2021) the South Africa variant is present in at least twenty states. The Pfizer-BioNTech vaccine is believed to be effective against the South Africa variant. There is indication that the Moderna and Pfizer-BioNTech vaccines might be effective against the UK variant.

The Brazilian variant may be the most elusive in terms of effectiveness of the current vaccines and may require a booster. All of the vaccine companies are working on follow-up boosters that may be administered in late 2021 to combat the predominant and concerning variants.

There will likely be ongoing coronavirus mutations, some of which will be more dangerous and more contagious, and some less so. In the end, news about any COVID mutations or variants should not affect our decision to receive the current COVID vaccine as soon as possible.

17. **To get back to your social life, restaurants, and gatherings**

The sooner we achieve and maintain the critically important herd immunity, the sooner we can return to normal life. I believe that we can have a nearly normal life of socializing, dining in restaurants, going to movies and parties, and traveling once we vaccinate a sizable percentage of the population. As we move forward, it's unrealistic to believe that life will be just as it was before the pandemic; there will be added screening, especially for large gatherings such as concerts.

The sooner our communities become vaccinated, the sooner we can get back to something approaching normal. One advantage of our situation is that, once we do return to normal, we will have a newfound knowledge of and appreciation for good hygiene, which will likely translate into the decline of infectious diseases in general. We can do most of the things that we did before, but we will have to be vigilant and perhaps do significantly more handwashing to avoid a repeat pandemic.

18. **To be able to travel safely**

For Thanksgiving 2020, my family, like most American families, elected to celebrate apart from our extended family. My family had a large Zoom Thanksgiving celebration, including my mother and father and my brothers' families. We each took turns describing what we missed most about our pre-pandemic lives, and many of us talked about travel that we missed throughout the year. My niece was especially melancholy over being prevented from visiting her friends last summer. Many of us have been going stir-crazy without our once- or twice-per-year vacation breaks.

Airports have devoted significant resources to making their facilities safer with social distancing and security lines. The airlines have upgraded their air circulation systems on planes, now recycling the air about every thirty seconds. Corporations are recommending that their employees get vaccinated before returning to work in offices and before traveling. Every holiday since the pandemic began, public health officials have worried about COVID spreading further. There was an uptick in COVID cases following both the Thanksgiving and Christmas holidays in 2020. To travel safely, it's important for the whole country–the whole world–to get vaccinated. Americans will not be permitted to visit countries with a lower incidence of COVID until we get our numbers under control, and the best way to do so is with widespread vaccination. Airlines in the states, at the time of this publication, are discussing the possibility of requiring proof of a negative COVID test or of a COVID vaccination before allowing people to board a plane.

19. To feel a sense of self-fulfillment that you did something for your fellow human beings

The feeling you get from making the choice to help bring hope to others in your community will change you. It will make you a better person and put you on a path to a more meaningful life. This is not an exaggeration. Getting vaccinated and encouraging others to get vaccinated will transform your community, making it more healthy, vibrant, and cohesive. Getting vaccinated is a powerful choice, perhaps one of the most powerful choices you can make to help end the pandemic and bring back hope.

Getting the vaccine is like volunteering or donating funds or resources to those in need—you are making a difference in the lives of others. Getting a COVID vaccine and helping us all get back to normal life is the best thing we can do right now to help others and ourselves.

By getting vaccinated and encouraging others to get vaccinated, you're helping create a better world for everyone. You are part of a collective public-health initiative, one that has a massive multiplier effect that will ripple throughout our country and the world. Besides preventing countless people from contracting and potentially dying from COVID, we can help hasten the opening of businesses and reduce unemployment. By getting the vaccine, you can feel a sense of fulfillment for helping to restore the world to better health, creating a world with the real human connectedness that we all crave.

8 TIPS ON HOW TO LIVE A HEALTHY, COVID-PREVENTIVE LIFESTYLE

"River cuts rock not because of its power, but its persistence."

— James N. Watkins

DEFEATING THE VIRUS REQUIRES THAT we build a set of key skills. One of these skills is day-to-day persistence in seeking to understand the virus and how to prevent it and in considering new information. When you're weak, lean on others who are stronger, and when you're stronger, give back to those who are wavering. For now, we cannot afford any weakness in our armor against the virus, and we must be persistent in our daily routines to prevent its spread. Many of us are suffering from COVID fatigue, but we must be relentlessly persistent. If we all do this for the length of time recommended by our public health officials, the number of cases and deaths will fall.

Here are my top ten tips on how to live a healthy, COVID-preventive lifestyle:

1. **Learn to love the mask**.

It is believed that mask wearing reduces an individual's risk of infection by 65 percent. Wearing a mask also prevents community spread of COVID. Be sure to choose a mask that is proven effective, is comfortable, and that maintains a tight seal over your nose, mouth, and chin. You should never touch the front of the mask, as it might be contaminated; touch only the loops on the back when putting the mask on or taking it off. Make sure the same side of the mask always faces outward. Always wash your hands before and after touching your mask. When you take off your mask, store it in a plastic bag. Cloth masks can be washed daily. Paper masks should be disposed of daily. Masks with valves do not provide protection. There will be times when mask wearing will become less needed and then we will revert back to wearing masks when infection occurs in a particular community. The above instructions are to be used when masks are recommended. Mask wearing should also be considered when you're in contact with those who have not been vaccinated or cannot be vaccinated because they are immunocompromised or have other serious health issues.

2. **Always carry sanitizer.**

The CDC recommends handwashing with soap and water for twenty seconds.

Handwashing reduces the amount and types of germs on the hands. If handwashing is not possible, then use a hand sanitizer with at least 60 percent alcohol. Handwashing is important because it reduces the amount of infection, sometimes significantly. It is estimated that handwashing and sanitizing decreases respiratory illnesses such as colds by about 20 percent and diarrheal diseases by about 30 percent. Handwashing at regular intervals is a must—after coughing or sneezing, after using the toilet, before eating, while preparing food, and after handling animals or animal waste. Be very mindful to wash hands after touching common surfaces, such as doorknobs and handles, and after returning home from visiting any public place. Don't forget to have a spare hand sanitizer in your car, purse, or backpack, and a few extra bottles at home.

3. **Move briskly through public places**.

Try not to stay in one place too long; keep moving, especially if you're in a smaller room for longer than fifteen minutes. Studies show that being in a room for fifteen minutes with someone who has COVID dramatically increases your risk of getting COVID. Use your best judgment before going out, and consider the current level of COVID-19 cases in the community.

4. **Avoid crowds.**

This practice is, of course, common sense. It takes only one asymp-tomatic person with COVID in a crowd to spread it to the whole crowd. Avoid people who do not avoid crowds.

5. **If you have to travel, travel safely**.

The CDC has identified a pattern of COVID surges following holi-day periods, when more people travel. If you don't need to travel, then don't do it until the numbers come down nationally, when the CDC can recommend travel. If you have to be inside airports, leave adequate time to move through the airport safely. If you can get hold of two N95 masks for your outbound and inbound journeys, this will protect you better in airports and on the plane than the standard surgical masks people wear.

6. **Strengthen your immune system**.

Practice a healthy lifestyle that supports strong immunity. Get at least seven hours of sleep every night. Getting seven hours of sleep is crucial for our immune systems to maintain their highest function. Eat whole, nutritious foods and fewer processed foods and snacks. Drink plenty of water. Exercise regularly, getting at least 150 minutes of moderate-intensity exercise per week. Stress can weaken your immunity, so have good support to help maintain your emotional well-being.

7. **Avoid immune-system zappers.**

Alcohol, cigarettes, vaping, and illicit drugs can compromise your immune system, making you more vulnerable to COVID-19. Avoid these things, especially if you have a preexisting condition that's already straining your immune system.

8. **Create a COVID-free social bubble or pod.**

Social pods help flatten the curve and prevent community spread. The goal of these groups is to allow us to socialize safely, which means you should still wear masks and socially distance during get-togethers with others who are living a COVID-safe lifestyle. Here are a few suggestions for creating a social pod: Limit your pod to about ten people or two to three households. It is recommended that the people in the pods be about the same age. Before starting a pod, make a list of agreed-upon rules, especially around touching and hugging. Set an understanding as to what will happen once someone is vaccinated and what to do if someone in the bubble gets sick. You must also agree on what to do when you're outside the bubble. It is recommended that everyone practice all of these rules for two weeks before the bubble starts. Once you form a social pod, you can also share COVID information to help the group and others avoid infection.

9. **Create vaccinated herds.**

Encourage your family, friends, and coworkers to get vaccinated so you can gather safely in person without fear of contracting COVID. If you spend time with ten people throughout the week and eight of them get the vaccine, it's very unlikely that those in your group will bring COVID to each other. Consistently encouraging each other to get vaccinated and to get the boosters that are likely to be offered in the future will prevent COVID from coming close to your group.

10. **Share reliable information**.

Reach out to your friends and family to share useful information, local updates, and inspiration. The most comprehensive web page for COVID-19 information is the Centers for Disease Control and Prevention site (cdc.gov). It has a variety of information on health and vaccines and updates in these categories. The health and vaccine sections will probably have the most useful information right now for most people. The health section has information about symptoms, including a symptom checker, and you can order posters about how to stop the spread of germs. The vaccine section has information about what to do before you get the vaccine, different groups getting the vaccine, and vaccine safety and monitoring. https://www.cdc.gov/coronavirus/2019-ncov/index.html

Another useful resource for updates on testing, treatments, and vaccines is the National Institutes of Health coronavirus web page: www.COVID19.nih.gov.

Finally, if you search Google news and type in COVID, you'll find updates on national and global cases and vaccines, along with links to other important stories.

COVID STRESS TIPS

The next four tips are to help with some very common COVID stressors that my patients have experienced. If you have any of these stressors, seek out a knowledgeable and empathetic clinician to help you through them.

1. COVID stressor number one: I think I have COVID

Here, I will offer my advice on how to calmly deal with each of these. For the stressor "I think I have COVID," it's important to recognize some of the common and some of the more severe symptoms of COVID. The common symptoms are dry cough, fever, shortness of breath, sore throat, headache, fatigue, and nausea. Lisa Maragakis, MD, MPH, senior director of infection prevention at Johns Hopkins, says, "It's important to distinguish between these common symptoms with other medical conditions." Your doctor or health care provider can distinguish COVID from other medical conditions. Don't try to diagnose COVID yourself. If you don't have a health care provider, it's a good time to get one. To decrease the stress level, it's important to contact a health care professional early on, so you don't spend time stressed out. They can reassure you quickly and tell you if you need to go for testing or wait it out.

2. **COVID stressor number two: I was just diagnosed with COVID and I am afraid**

It's completely natural to be afraid of a COVID diagnosis. I have diagnosed hundreds of cases of COVID and there's usually a similar scenario when my patient's test is positive. First, they feel somewhat guilty about contracting it. I tell them COVID is very infectious, it's easy to get, don't be hard on yourself that you got COVID. I tell them when we get the flu and are sick at home for a while, we just get over it and move on with our life and don't worry about how we got it, nor do we stigmatize people who get the flu. Next, they're worried about the course of COVID. I reassure them by telling them when to call me when severe symptoms develop. Finally, they worry about going back to work or normal life. Most of the persistent symptoms like cough and lack of taste and smell persist a lot longer than the standard ten days that you can be infective. I end up speaking to these patients a little more often throughout the week to make sure their symptoms clear and they are headed in the right direction.

3. COVID stressor number three: I am afraid life will never be the same because of COVID

A recent survey from the American Psychological Association found that 49 percent of adults reported feeling uncomfortable about returning to in-person interactions when the pandemic ends. Even 48 percent of those who received the vaccine reported feeling that way. During the lockdown and right afterwards, many of my patients were overly pessimistic about the situation and thought we would never get out of the pandemic. I reassured them that with the public health measures we were taking and with the vaccine, we would get back to a new normal. We have to recognize that some of the anxiety is due to the uncertainty of when things will get back to normal, and we must accept this degree of uncertainty. We must also understand that from being at home for so long, we may have a degree of social anxiety, and we have to plan and take baby steps and get out of our homes in a safe way.

4. COVID stressor number four: I had COVID a long time ago and I still have symptoms

Most people recover from COVID in two to six weeks. Researchers have found that some take months to recover from COVID and are calling this condition "long COVID" or "post-COVID syndrome." A term that some are using to refer to themselves is "COVID long-haulers." My patients are stressed because they're not certain if this is a result of having COVID or something else. The best way for you to cope with this stress is to give a detailed history to your doctor and be open to having tests run to determine other causes of the symptoms. The symptoms of long COVID, including fatigue, confusion, headache, joint pain, and fever, which may come and go, also occur in many other diagnoses. There's often intense physical and psychological stress with a diagnosis of COVID, so it's important to understand that both your body and your mind have gone through this stress and need time to recover. Set realistic goals for your life and work during this recovery period. Try to get more rest and relaxation.

9 MOVING TOWARD A HEALTHIER, BETTER INFORMED POST-COVID WORLD

"In the rush to get back to normal, use time to decide which parts of normal are worth rushing back to."

– Dave Hollis

EARLIER, I MENTIONED FALSE NEWS items about COVID and debunked them. It is my hope that we will be more vigilant about demonstrably false health news, because it really does affect our health. This has been magnified during the COVID pandemic, when not doing the right thing really did lead directly to people suffering and dying. I can give you some general guidelines about how to separate fact from fiction, the best websites to consult, and other tips for avoiding false health news.

Since March 2020, I've given many lectures in rehab and nursing facilities on what COVID is, identifying the symptoms, explaining how to protect patients, and, of course, explaining and promoting

COVID vaccines. I've given countless lectures over the past twenty years, primarily to nurses, empowering them to think critically and communicate more effectively with doctors. During my recent COVID lectures, the nurses' attention has been more acute. They are curious, and they ask more questions because some of these issues have already impacted them, and they want to learn how to protect themselves and their patients.

I take it upon myself to actively debunk conspiracy theories and medical myths. The truth is that medical misinformation doesn't just lead to misunderstanding—it can kill you. I am encouraged that people are addressing conspiracy theories they hear about on social media by seeking out more authoritative sites and dispelling the myths on their own.

It was not until the measles epidemic in early 2019 that the imperative to root out fake medical news was taken seriously. When the COVID pandemic began, the mainstream media started addressing these medical myths in a more responsible way. YouTube, Facebook, and Pinterest all began addressing them in 2019 and are now doing so even more. COVID has accelerated this process so that we can uncover the truth regarding COVID more quickly and perhaps, in the future, regarding other medical conditions as well.

Since the start of the pandemic, it appears that we are coming to an informed world and people are turning to trusted health websites.

More people have been introduced to websites that are more reliable. Traffic on cdc.gov, for example, has increased dramatically.

Better hygiene techniques, such as using hand sanitizer, covering your mouth when you sneeze, and not touching your face, have resulted in lower transmission of influenza A and B, along with other respiratory and gastrointestinal (GI) infectious diseases, in 2020 and 2021. I believe that these habits will also translate to fewer infectious diseases after we defeat COVID.

Current dramatic advances in vaccine development and a greater acceptance of vaccines, along with the rebuilding of local and state public health departments, will translate to a healthier population in the future. From volunteering for food drives to checking on elderly neighbors to replacing the goodbye salutation with "be safe," COVID has brought out a new level of common caring and compassion in us, which I believe will continue in the post-COVID world, thereby creating a healthier nation and a healthier world.

ABOUT THE AUTHOR

DOMINIC GAZIANO, M.D. - DR G., as his patients know him - is the director of Body and Mind Medical Center based in Chicago, Il. In his practice, he brings together holistic, researched-based therapeutic strategies from both eastern and western medicine.

Dr. Gaziano has been in the trenches of American healthcare two immensely turbulent decades. Dr. G. believes that your doctor can help you on your journey of self-health and happiness by helping you understand how your life stresses impact your life and health. Dr. Gaziano has authored 3 other books, "Feel Good Health," a seasonal health and wellness tips guide; "Well Now!," a more comprehensive strategy for your self-health as well as Dr. G.'s insight in dealing with various healthcare systems challenges; "A Doctor's Cure for Medical Myths," where he debunks common medical misinformation.

He regularly gives lectures, seminars, and destination retreats on resilience and stress management. Dr. G. has been a local and national television and radio commentator on current various medical topics such as COVID, the opioid epidemic and vaping.

For more information visit www.dominicgazianomd.com.

ACKNOWLEDGMENTS

Al Pak for the amazing Illustrations

Kathy Meis and Shilah LaCoe of Bublish who helped keep me on track on the sometimes arduous book journey with great advice and motivation

www.ingramcontent.com/pod-product-compliance
Lightning Source LLC
Chambersburg PA
CBHW071436210326
41597CB00020B/3811